Finding & Choosing a Safe and Quality Nail Salon

The Complete Guide to Nail Care

TIFFANIE LEE

Acknowledgments

I want to thank my husband, Leng Lee, for the faith that he has in me writing this book. I would not be able to get my book done without his continual support and understanding of my vision. He was there from reading early draft to helping me with formatting.

Erin Lyman, my editor and proofreader, for editing and proofreading.

My friend, Debra Wiseman, for reviewing the final draft.

To God for most of all, because of him, all the impossible was possible.

Contents

Preface

In 2015, I made a big leap and decided to open a nail salon. It was located in a trendy downtown area with many boutique shops, restaurants, small businesses, and a few beauty salons. Clients loved our work and how clean the salon was. Beauty salon owners and their employees even came to us for their nail services and recommended us to their clients. It was a very successful nail salon. Its reputation far exceeded what I had expected when I first opened the nail salon.

When the pandemic hit in 2020, the nail salon had to close in the middle of March and did not reopen until August. Once it reopened, it was difficult to get the nail technicians to come back to work. This was a common problem in other nail salons, as well. The nail technicians who did come back to work were not able to keep a set schedule due to COVID, sickness, childcare, or other reasons. This caused many nail appointments to be canceled or rescheduled. Despite this, our clients were very understanding.

In addition, the prices of nail products skyrocketed due to shortages. For example, a pair of gloves that used to cost twenty-five cents were now two or three dollars per pair, depending on the size. My nail product distributors were having a hard time sourcing nail products. Every time I placed an order, I was lucky if I received half of what I ordered.

Due to these difficulties, I decided to close the nail salon in the summer of 2021. It was not an easy decision, the salon and employees were like family to me. In the fall of 2021, I decided to rent a salon suite closer to home after reading many sad, frustrated, and disappointed emails from my clients about their experiences at other nail salons.

Once I opened the salon suite, my clients came back and told me about their nail horror stories. Many of them asked me what they should be looking for when choosing a nail salon. I shared my knowledge with all of them, and now would like to share it with all of you. I hope this book will help make it easier for you to know what to look for when searching for a safe and quality nail salon, and hopefully to find the perfect one.

Chapter One

Knowing What You Need

Have you ever walked into a nail salon with high expectations only to leave disappointed? Maybe the service wasn't up to par, or what you expected. That's why it's crucial to understand what you need before you start looking for a nail salon. When you take the time to understand what you need, it will help you narrow down the nail salons that may be the right fit for you. Three topics I find most useful when trying to understand your needs are lifestyle, budget, and special occasion.

LIFESTYLE

What's your lifestyle like? Are you always on the go, or do you have a lot of free time? If you're busy, you may want a quick and simple service. If you have more time, you may want a relaxing and luxurious experience.

BUDGET

Prices vary depending on services and from salon to salon. Ask yourself, "How much am I willing to spend on a nail service?" Knowing your budget can help you find a nail salon that fits your budget.

SPECIAL OCCASION

Are you getting your nails done for a special event, or are you just looking to pamper yourself? If you're getting your nails done for a special event, you may want a more elaborate service. If you're just looking to pamper yourself, you may want a simple and relaxing service.

After you know what you need, you will need to prioritize those needs. For example, if you're looking for a nail salon that fits your budget and is environmentally friendly, you can prioritize that when searching for a salon. Or, if you're looking for a salon that offers high-quality products, you can prioritize that as well. By prioritizing your needs, you can find a salon that best aligns with your values and provides the service you need.

It's also important to remember that everyone's needs are different. What may be important to you may not be important to someone else. That's why it's essential to take the time to assess your needs.

Chapter Two

Finding A Nail Salon

There are many sources to help you find a nail salon, but I find that only four are really useful. Knowing what to look for when using these sources will give you more confidence when choosing a nail salon. You will also feel more relaxed when entering into a nail salon you have never been to, and you will be able to enjoy the experience.

ONLINE REVIEWS

Imagine you are going to attend a wedding this weekend and need to have your nails done. You start Googling nail salons in your area and start reading their reviews on Yelp or Google, but how do you really know if the salons are any good?

Online reviews from Yelp, Facebook, and Google are very useful resources when it comes to finding a trustworthy nail salon. A good review includes enough detail to give others a feel for what happened. Explain which factors contributed to their positive, negative, or just so-so experience. Reviews will give you a general idea of what the salon is like.

When reading reviews, pay very close attention to what the review is about. Typically, the review will either be about the nail service or customer service experience. You want to focus on bad nail service reviews. An example of a bad nail service review is when a client received an acrylic set that was supposed to last up to three weeks but lifted in three days, or a manicure in which cuticles were excessively trimmed which caused bleeding. Too many bad nail service reviews are a sign that the nail salon may not be for you.

Next, see if the salon responds to any bad reviews. This will give you an idea of how the salon is managed. You want to know how proactive they are in addressing complaints by clients. The salon responses to reviews should be helpful, rather than argumentative. If you read the reviews and find the complaints are very similar then the salon may not be a good fit for you.

TRIP TO THE SALON

Walk in and take a quick look around the salon. When you chat with the receptionist, sneak a peek at the display wall. Do you see any certificates issued by the government for the salon or nail technicians? The government wants you to know that your nail technician is licensed to do your nails.

The number of certificates should match the number of nail technicians working in the salon. If it doesn't, that's a major red flag.

When it comes to picking a nail salon, safety and cleanliness should be your top priorities. Don't be afraid to ask questions and observe your surroundings.

PRICE AND LENGTH OF SERVICE

The old adage, "You get what you pay for," rings true in the nail industry. Be wary of nail salons that advertise acrylic sets, no chip manicure, or mani/pedi combo for a ridiculously low price. Usually they are cutting corners and using cheap, inferior products.

Length of service may vary from place to place but should not vary greatly. It should take at least forty-five minutes for a licensed, experienced nail technician to finish a no-chip manicure service and at least one hour with removal if the client's nails still have old nail polish on. In our salon, we take our time to do each service (one hour and fifteen minutes for a no chip manicure with removal, and two hours for an acrylic or dip powder set).

There were so many times when a nail technician or I finished a service and the client would make a comment like, "What a big difference between a thirty minute vs one hour manicure." Yes, that is right! A beautiful, long lasting manicure requires a lot of attention to detail. Twenty to thirty minutes is not enough to do a full manicure service plus removal.

Most salons have online booking now. You can check the price and length of service by going to their booking website.

RECOMMENDATIONS

Ask your friends and family members for a recommendation. It is also one of the very best ways to find a good nail salon to go to. I remember doing a dip powder service for a client who drove almost three hours to come to see me. Her college friend came to visit her. Coincidentally, she and her friend both happened to have the same dip powder color that day, but she said she thought her friend's nails looked so much more beautiful than hers. She asked her friend who did it. Her friend told her it was done by me and that was why she drove all the way to see me.

Another way is to ask your co-workers at your workplace. Young professionals love to get their nails done. They do it every two to three weeks, so they know good places to go. Many clients told me they heard about my nail salon from co-workers at work.

Do not be afraid to ask if you see someone with beautiful nails. People love it when you compliment their nails. My clients always tell me which color they got the most compliments from. They may tell you who they see if you ask, so don't be shy.

Now you have the information to help you find a nail salon that you will like to go to. Let us talk about other things that you have to consider such as cleanliness and sanitation, licensing, and type of nail technicians, in order to help you narrow your choices.

Chapter Three
Cleanliness and Sanitation

Cleanliness and sanitation are the two of the most critical factors when it comes to nail salons. When it comes to choosing a nail salon, you need to consider how clean and sanitary the salon is. No one wants to go to a nail salon that is dirty or unsafe.

CLEANLINESS

Cleanliness is not just important for aesthetic purposes; it's also essential for your health and safety. A clean nail salon indicates that the staff cares about their customers' well-being and takes pride in their work. A dirty or disorganized salon can be a breeding ground for germs and bacteria, which can lead to infections and other health issues. Therefore, it's crucial to find a nail salon that prioritizes cleanliness and maintains a clean environment.

SANITATION

Sanitation is crucial, yet it's often overlooked. It's not just about the physical appearance of the salon. Sanitation goes beyond a clean surface or a fresh scent. It's about the safety of the customers. Unsanitary conditions can lead to infections, diseases, and even permanent damage to your nails and skin.

Don't compromise your health and well-being for a pretty polish job. Choose a salon that prioritizes sanitation and safety. Your nails and feet will thank you in the long run.

Why is sanitation so important? Proper sanitation prevents the spread of fungal and bacterial diseases from one client to another and helps to ensure safe working conditions in the salon.

What does proper sanitation mean?

- Clean all work areas, manicure stations, and pedicure stations after each client.

- Wipe down and vacuum debris such as nail pieces or nail dust after every service.

- Always use clean towel for each client.

- Use a new nail file, buffer, and pumice stone for each client as these are made of materials that are porous and cannot be sanitized, disinfected, or sterilized.

- Sanitize, disinfect, sterilize, and package all metal implements. However, many states do not require nail salons to sterilize their metal implements such as nail clippers, pushers, and nippers.

Other good sanitary practices are:

- Have nail technicians wear gloves at all times when performing a service.

- Have nail technicians wash their hands between clients. It is also better to use liquid hand soap than bar soap when washing your hands and using paper towels to dry your hands.

- Do not share anything that was used. It is not sanitary. I remember my hair instructor once said, "Treat everyone that comes in the door as if they have a disease, because you just never know."

- Have clients wash their hands before a manicure, and soak their feet before a pedicure.

I cannot stress enough the importance of prioritizing safety over beauty when choosing a nail salon. Your nails may seem like a small aspect of your overall health, but they are not to be overlooked. And let's be honest, who doesn't want to walk out of a salon with gorgeous nails? But at what cost? Choosing a salon solely based on their ability to create stunning nail designs can lead to serious health consequences. Nail salons that cut corners, when it comes to sanitation practices, put their clients at risk for infections and diseases. It's not only uncomfortable but can also lead to more serious health issues.

Your nails are a reflection of your overall health, and it's important to take care of them properly. Remember, beauty fades, but your health should always be a priority. It's better to be safe than sorry!

Chapter Four

Licensed Nail Technician

Every state requires a license to be a nail salon technician, although there are different nail technician licensing requirements in each state. All states require a certain amount of education, training in a cosmetology or nail technician program, and passing a test to receive a nail technician license. This is a way of ensuring that every nail technician is equipped with the knowledge and skills to make your nails look and feel amazing.

It's also worth noting that a licensed nail technician in one state cannot work in another state without obtaining a license in that state. This ensures that they are following the specific guidelines and regulations of each state, which is crucial when it comes to maintaining high standards of hygiene and safety.

Why do you want a licensed nail technician to do your nails?

- Professionalism: When you visit a licensed nail technician, you can be confident that you are working with a professional who has undergone extensive training and has the necessary qualifications to provide safe and effective nail care services.

- Safety: Licensed nail technicians are required to follow strict safety and sanitation protocols to prevent the spread of infections and other health risks. This includes using clean and properly sanitized tools and equipment, as well as following best nail care practices.

- Quality: When you work with a licensed nail technician, you can be assured that you are receiving high-quality nail care services. These professionals are held to a high standard of excellence and are committed to providing the best possible care to their clients.

- Peace of Mind: Working with a licensed and insured nail technician gives you peace of mind that you are in good hands. If anything should go wrong during your appointment, you can be confident that your technician has the necessary insurance to cover any damages or injuries.

If the nail technician you see is not licensed, DON'T BE SURPRISED! But here's the thing: going to an unlicensed nail technician can be risky. These individuals may not have gone through the necessary education, training, and testing to provide quality services. They may not know how to properly sanitize their tools or be aware of the latest nail trends.

At the end of the day, it's important to do your research and choose a salon with licensed technicians. This ensures that you're getting quality services from professionals who know what they're doing. Plus, it's a way of supporting those who have put in the time and effort to become certified in their field.

In my experience, many licensed nail technicians eventually want to work for themselves. They enjoy the freedom of being their own boss and creating their own schedules. And who can blame them? It's a great feeling to have that kind of independence and control over your work. But that can make it even harder for customers to find a licensed nail technician they like. It's like trying to find a needle in a haystack sometimes! That's why, when you do find a licensed nail technician you love, hold on to them tightly. Cherish them and their skills, and make sure to recommend them to your friends and family.

Chapter Five

Types of Nail Techs

There are three types of nail technicians that you will most likely encounter. Knowing the differences will help you make an easier decision. Before we start listing the types of nail technicians and the pros and the cons, I'd like to share my story.

I remember the first nail salon I ever worked for. I went to the interview and was hired on the spot. They told me to come back the next day to start working. I thought they might provide training when I showed up the next day. On my first day on the job, I was told to take clients all day. I had no idea where the tools were, what the procedures were (if there were any), how to set up, or where to turn on the water on the pedicure chair. I was basically clueless. I was expecting some training like when I first finished cosmetology school and went to work at a hair salon, but that was not the case. I was never good at what I did while I worked there. Clients would come back for fixes all the time and sometimes I knew about it, but most of the time the complaints were handled by someone at the front desk. The worst part was when I found out that I was an independent contractor nail technician and not an employee, which I thought I was. It's a good thing that I only worked there for a month. This is why it is important to know what type of nail technician you go to.

TYPE #1 – EMPLOYEE

A nail technician working under the direction of a nail salon is an employee of the salon. They are hired by the salon to provide nail care services to the salon's clients and receive a regular paycheck with taxes withheld. The salon will provide the tools, supplies, and equipment needed to perform the job. The salon sets the work hours and pricing of services as well as provides training and policies. Nail technicians may have limited control over their schedule, price, and service offerings. The quality and cleanliness in the salon is controlled by the employer. The nail technicians who work as employees are insured by the employer.

Nail salons who have employees usually would pair the newly hired employee with a senior nail technician to shadow for a day or so before letting him or her start taking clients. For most salons like these and mine, they usually would have the newly-hired employee bring in a model to work on to show his or her skills. This way the salon knows what areas to train the newly-hired employee.

Pros: Quality of nail service is very consistent. Appointment will be on time. There is always someone that you can address your complaint. Nail technicians are insured. Nail technicians are up to date with nail trends and state protocols.

Cons: Nail technicians do not stay long at one salon. They tend to move from one salon to another. No one will let you know where your favorite nail technician went.

TYPE #2 – INDEPENDENT CONTRACTOR

A nail technician who signs a contract to work for a nail salon for a period of time without the direction of the nail salon and receives no training, even if they just finished school, is an independent contractor. They perform nail services using their own methods or what they know. They are responsible for their own tools, nail products (some nail salons will provide nail polishes), and equipment. They will also set their own prices and service offerings. But do not be surprised if everyone is charged the same.

The nail technician is responsible for sanitizing, disinfecting and sterilizing their own tools, and cleaning their work station. They are responsible for their work and any injuries that may occur during and after the service. They may have more control over their schedule and the services they provide, but they have to pay their own taxes and buy their own liability insurance. The salon or spa may charge him or her a fee to use their space or take a percentage of their earnings as commission.

Pros: Walk-Ins are readily available. Each service is done fast. Easy to get an appointment.

Cons: Quality of service is different each time, depending on who you see. Expect to wait a little longer even when you have an appointment. The nail salon will not be responsible if anything should go wrong.

TYPE #3 – BOOTH RENTER

A booth renter nail technician is someone who rents a space at a salon suite to operate their own nail care business. They are responsible for all aspects of their business, including setting their own prices, providing their own supplies and equipment, and managing their own schedule.

They have one hundred percent control over their business operations. They are responsible for paying their own taxes, liability insurance (some salon suites provide liability insurance for their renters), and rent for their space.

Usually, booth renters are nail technicians who have many years of experience in the field and have lots of clientele already.

Pros: Service quality is consistent. You have more privacy. Nail technician is skilled and knowledgeable.

Cons: Hard to get an appointment. You have to schedule your appointment weeks ahead. You do not have anyone else to see if your nail technician takes vacation or is sick.

Each of these types of nail technician providers have their own advantages and disadvantages, and it is important to consider which option is best for your individual situation. Regardless of which type of provider you choose, it is important to choose a skilled and experienced technician who can provide the high-quality nail care services you deserve.

As for me, I would prefer to see a nail technician that works for a salon as an employee because he or she is insured, trained, and licensed. The service will usually be on time. And if anything goes wrong or the service was sub-par, I know who to go to with my complaint.

Chapter Six

Words of Advice

I would like to share some words of advice from my experience as a nail salon owner.

LISTEN TO YOUR NAIL PROFESSIONAL

We live in a world where the Internet is available to everyone. You can find just about anything you would like to know with just a touch of your finger. Do not always assume that the information you find on the web is accurate. I found out many times that it was not. Listen to your nail technician when he or she advises you on your nail care. There is a reason your nail technician is licensed. If he or she advises you to take a break, take a break! It is good for your nails.

A couple of years ago, I had two clients who came to see us. One was the mom and the other was her daughter. I did the daughter's nails, and one of my employees did the mom's nails. Both of their nails were very thin. Both of them had done acrylic nails for years. The mom told me she read on the Internet that dip powder will help their thin nails get thicker and longer. The mom's friend, who is a client of ours, recommended us to her because of our excellent dip powder service. The mom liked the fact that we do not *dip*, but we *pour*, and that is why she came to see us. I hated to disappoint her, but I had to tell her the truth, that the information she read was incorrect.

No nail products will heal nails that are broken, thin, fragile, or brittle. It is meant to enhance the look of your nails. Cosmetics are made to beautify only.

COMMUNICATE WITH YOUR NAIL PROFESSIONAL

It's important to communicate what you want to the nail salon staff, so they can provide the service that is best for you. For example, if you want a simple manicure, you can communicate that to the staff, and they can provide the service accordingly. On the other hand, if you want a luxury spa pedicure, they can offer that as well.

Also, let your nail professional know if you have any health or nail issues. This way your nail professional will know what to do and how to take care of you.

CALLUSES AND CUTICLES

I would like to discuss more about calluses and cuticles. I feel these two topics are most misunderstood by clients.

A callus is a rough, thick layers of skin. It develops because of repeated pressure or irritation of the skin and usually found on the palms of the hand and soles of the feet. When clients come to get their pedicure done, some will ask us to use a cheese grater and I tell them, "No, not in my salon." Calluses are our skin's natural defense mechanism. Calluses only need to be smooth and softened by using a pumice stone. If the calluses are severe enough that it requires removal, your nail technician will refer you to a podiatrist. Nail technicians are limited in removing calluses. By removing it, it can cause other problems. Cheese graters are illegal to use to scrape calluses in many states. Listen to your nail technician if he or she says you do not need it or advises you to go to see a doctor.

Cuticles are the layer of clear dead skin on the surface of the nail plate. Since this tissue is dead, most of it can be safely trimmed. Do not ask your nail technician to trim your cuticle more than what he or she thinks is needed. Excessive trimming of the cuticles could result in bleeding and increases the development of hangnails around your nails. The most difficult part to learn when doing a manicure or pedicure is trimming cuticles. It is very scary but it is an important step that will make your nails beautiful.

Again, ALWAYS LISTEN TO YOUR NAIL TECHNICIAN. I can not emphasize how important this is.

KEEP YOUR NAILS STRONG AND HEALTHY WHEN AT HOME

Have you ever stopped to think about how important your nails are? Not only do they serve as a canvas for fun nail art and polish colors, but they can also be a reflection of your overall health. Always keep in mind your nails are jewels not tools. Here is a list of things to keep your nails strong and healthy when at home:

- Do not use them to open soda cans and anything that can break them.

- Never peel off your no-chip gel polishes or any nail enhancements that were put on your nails. Go to see your nail technician and have it done properly to avoid damaging the nail plates.

- Eat foods that are good for your nails and hair.

- Ask your doctor about taking nail and hair supplements.

- Always remember to wear gloves when washing dishes, as water and chemicals like detergents can leave your nails weak, dull, and brittle.

- Massage cuticle oil into the nails, cuticles, and the skin around the nail daily to give some strength and flexibility. This is best done at night when you do not have to wash your hands frequently.

- Do not bite your nails or pick your hangnails. Many clients told me the reason they get their nails done every two to three weeks was because they have a habit of biting and picking on their nails.

Prolonged nail biting and picking can lead to a painful, red, swollen inflammation around the nail, or at the site of the hangnail.

Chapter Seven
Nail Horror Stories

Working in the nail salon, you hear a lot of nail horror stories from your clients. I would like to share with you several stories that clients told us in my salon.

Horror Story #1

A young lady walked into my salon for an acrylic removal, I could tell she was embarrassed and ashamed of her nails. Before I could even take a look, she apologized profusely for their terrible condition. As I examined her nails, my heart sank. Her acrylics had been on for far too long, and the damage was evident. The tips were half-broken, the acrylics were lifting and cracking all over the nail plates, and some of her natural nails were broken in half, with dried blood still present. The smell was overwhelming, and it was evident that something was seriously wrong.

I recommended that she see a medical doctor right away, explaining that a nail technician cannot treat anything that needs medical attention. It was clear that her nails needed more than just a simple removal and a new set of enhancements. My heart went out to her, and I couldn't help but feel frustrated and angry that nobody had told her the consequences of neglecting her nails.

When I asked her why she didn't get it fixed when she first noticed the lifting and cracking of the enhancements, her response broke my heart even more. She simply didn't know that it would cause such severe problems because nobody had told her. It's moments like these that remind me of the importance of education and awareness when it comes to nail care. Neglecting your nails can have serious consequences, and it's up to us as professionals to educate our clients and provide them with the knowledge they need to take care of their nails properly.

So, if you're experiencing any issues with your nails, please seek help right away. Don't wait until it's too late, because the consequences can be severe.

Horror Story #2

A client who recently relocated from another city came for a dip powder service. She told me a few weeks ago that she went to a local nail salon for a dip powder service. As she waited in the waiting area to see her nail technician, she saw a nail technician (who was doing a dip powder service) take out a tissue from the manicure drawer and wipe the blood off from the client's nail. After wiping the blood off, the nail technician continued the service by dipping the client's fingers into the dip powder jar. She was a little nervous after seeing that.

A few minutes later, the lady at the front desk told her that her nail technician was ready to see her and directed her to a manicure table. She sat down and looked at the nail technician and realized it was the same nail technician that was using the tissue to wipe the last client's blood. She was more nervous now, but she went ahead with the service. However, she could not stop thinking about it the whole entire time.

When she got home, she told her husband the entire experience, but that did not make her feel any better. She decided to remove the dip powder herself, so she went to the drug store and bought alcohol and pure acetone. Even after the dip powder was removed, she still did not feel it was clean enough.

In my salon, we put a portion of the dip powder into a tiny dish. When the nails are finished prepping, we sprinkle or pour the dip powder over the nails. Dipping the nails into a jar of dip powder is not sanitary. I will tell you why. At least fifty percent of our clients who come to get their nails done have open wounds, scratches, or bleeding cuticles on their fingernails. By dipping the nails into the jar, it will contaminate the powder in the jar. So, look for a nail salon who only *pours*, not *dips*, when applying the powder onto your nails. Again, your nails are part of your overall health, do not forget that!

HORROR STORY #3

On a busy Saturday afternoon, a client came to the salon begging to have her one nail enhancement removed, but there was no nail technician available at the time, including myself. She started to cry. I came to the front desk to take a look at her finger. Her fingernail was red and almost purple. The skin around it was also red and swollen. I asked if she had bumped her nail against something, and she replied, "No". She said she just had her nails done five days ago. I asked her when she first felt the pain. She replied, "Last night." She did not know why it was hurting so badly, but she needed it to be removed and did not want to go back to the nail salon that did the enhancement.

I asked her to have a seat while I figured out our schedule. After about ten minutes I was able to see her. I removed the acrylic nail enhancement from her finger and noticed a split in the middle of the natural nail plate. I asked if that split was there when the enhancement was put on, and she said yes. She said the nail technician patched the split with glue and then put the acrylic on top. In the first few days, it was okay but on the fifth day, it started to bother her. I advised her to see a medical doctor.

This kind of treatment for nail splitting should not be done in the nail salon. Moisture can get trapped inside the split or nail bed which could lead to further problems down the road. In addition, it is outside the scope of what nail technicians are allowed to do. Only a medical doctor can treat something like that.

HORROR STORY # 4

A regular client of ours who came every month for her pedicure expressed how grateful she was to have found us after experiencing a bad pedicure service a couple of years ago. She said the nail technician used a cheese grater to scrape her calluses. The nail technician scraped so hard that one of her heels was bleeding. Blood was all over in the pedicure basin and the water turned pink, but the nail technician continued the service as if nothing was wrong. Nor did she apologize to her. She had to tell the nail technician to stop the service. After that experience, she stopped getting pedicures done until she found us on Yelp.

I do not approve the use of the cheese grater on clients' feet, and I prohibit the use in my salon. They are considered a banned item in salons in many states because it cannot only injure the client but also spread infection.

HORROR STORY #5

A client who I saw only one time said she had acrylic nails done all the time in the nineties. Every two to three weeks she would go to get them filled. But there were times that the acrylics had to be soaked off. The nail technician would remove the acrylics by soaking her hands with pure acetone in either a small bowl or plastic bag. The pure acetone covered her fingers all the way to the first knuckles. As the years went by, the cuticles became very dry. It got worse in the winter, and since then she stopped doing acrylic nails and any other nail service that had to do with acetone.

After we were done with the consultation, I decided to give her a nail service that did not use acetone. She wanted to see me again, but due to schedule conflicts, I paired her up with a senior nail technician who has been in my salon for many years.

Excessive use of acetone on the skin is not recommended.

HORROR STORY # 6

Another time in my salon, I overheard a new client telling one of my nail technicians about her no-chip manicure experience from a different nail salon. The client said she liked the technique my nail technician used to remove her old no-chip polishes. It did not hurt. The place where she went to before always used an electric nail file to file off her old no-chip polishes, and it would hurt a lot.

When she asked the nail technician if there was another way to remove the polishes without the electric nail file, the nail technician said, "No, this way is faster and better." Over the years, her nail plates became very thin.

Every nail technician has an electric nail file, but without proper training it can be misused. Faster and better may not be beneficial to the client in the long run. Also, the nail technician should listen to what the client is telling him or her. If it hurts, it hurts!

HORROR STORY # 7

I remember one particular client who just got her nails done by one of my nail technicians. I gave her a "DO and DON'T DO" pamphlet to read when she checked out. She said to me, "I don't need it. I've been getting my nails done for many years. I know all about it." She paid and left without the pamphlet.

When she returned a few months later, her fingernails were green. She told me she had her nails done somewhere else. The nail technician she saw always just filed it off and put a new set on. It has been that way for many years. She did not think it was anything serious.

I explained to her that when nail enhancements lift or crack, water could get inside the space between the nail plates and the enhancements. It needs to be fixed or removed, otherwise it could lead to bigger problems. I recommended that she see a doctor, and when it cleared up she could come back. She came back a couple months later with healthy nails and became a regular client until she relocated to a different state.

Nail enhancements are strong and can trap moisture inside if you don't get them fixed. When wearing nail enhancements, please pay close attention to your nails. If you notice any lifting, cracking, peeling, or breaking, do not try to fix it yourself. You need to call the nail salon and go back to get it fixed as soon as possible to avoid further problems.

Our nail salon had denied many nail services for customers who walked in with discolored fingernails. Some customers were not happy that they were denied, but for some, they got curious and asked to know more. Once they knew the reasons behind it, they were glad we denied their nail services and later made our salon a place for their nail care.